DR ROBERT CLARKSON

The Kidney Disease Solution

A Comprehensive Guide to Managing and Reversing
Chronic Kidney Disease

Contents

Introduction

It was a typical day for Frank. He was a retired accountant and enjoyed a peaceful life until he received a call from his doctor. The news was not good; he had been diagnosed with chronic kidney disease.

Frank was devastated. He had always taken care of his health, but now his doctor was telling him that his kidneys were failing and he needed to make lifestyle changes or face serious consequences.

Frank was determined to learn more about his condition and how to manage it. He searched the internet and soon came across The Kidney Disease Solution, a comprehensive guide to managing and reversing chronic kidney disease.

The guide was written by a team of medical professionals and provided detailed information on everything from the causes of kidney disease to treatment options and lifestyle changes he could make.

The guide also had sections devoted to diet and nutrition, exercise, and stress management. Frank was amazed at how much the guide had to offer and was inspired to make the necessary lifestyle changes to improve his health.

He followed the advice in the guide and within a few months, his health had improved significantly. His kidney function had improved, his energy levels had increased, and he felt better than ever.

Frank was overjoyed. He was so thankful to have found The Kidney Disease

Solution and for the life-saving advice it provided. He was now on the road to recovery and was feeling better than ever. Frank was grateful for the comprehensive guide and the positive changes it had made in his life.

He was also proud to have taken control of his health and to have been able to manage and reverse his chronic kidney disease. Thanks to The Kidney Disease Solution, Frank was finally free from the worry and stress of his condition.

He was now living a healthier, happier life and was looking forward to a brighter future.

1

Chapter 1

Overview of kidney function and anatomy

Sure, the kidneys are a pair of organs located in the back of the abdomen that are responsible for filtering waste products from the blood and regulating electrolyte balance. They are vital to overall health and play an important role in maintaining homeostasis in the body.

The kidneys are bean-shaped organs, each measuring about the size of a fist. They are located on either side of the spine, just below the rib cage. The right kidney is slightly lower than the left kidney due to the position of the liver.

The kidneys are composed of several structures, including the renal cortex and renal medulla. The renal cortex is the outer layer of the kidney and is responsible for producing hormones that regulate blood pressure and red blood cell production. The renal medulla is the inner layer of the kidney and is responsible for filtering waste products from the blood.

The kidneys filter waste products from the blood through millions of small filters called nephrons. Each nephron consists of a glomerulus (a ball of capillaries) and a tubule. Blood enters the glomerulus and waste products are filtered out into the tubule. The tubule then reabsorbs important substances, such as glucose and electrolytes, back into the bloodstream.

The renal artery carries oxygenated blood to the kidneys, while the renal vein carries deoxygenated blood away from the kidneys. The renal artery branches into smaller arteries that supply blood to the individual nephrons. The filtered blood exits the kidneys via the renal vein and returns to the heart.

The kidneys also play an important role in regulating electrolyte balance by filtering and reabsorbing electrolytes such as sodium and potassium. They also produce hormones, such as erythropoietin, which stimulates red blood cell production, and renin, which helps regulate blood pressure. Additionally, the kidneys produce active forms of vitamin D, which is vital for maintaining healthy bones.

The kidneys also work closely with other organs to maintain balance in the body. For example, they help regulate the balance of water and salt in the body, in coordination with the hormone aldosterone produced by the adrenal gland. In addition to this, it work with the parathyroid hormone to maintain the balance of calcium and phosphorus, which is important for bone health.

In addition to their role in maintaining homeostasis, the kidneys also play a critical role in the elimination of toxins and waste products from the body. They do this by filtering waste products, such as urea and creatinine, out of the blood and into the urine. The urine is then eliminated from the body through the ureters, bladder, and urethra.

However, when the kidneys are not functioning properly, these waste products can build up in the blood, leading to a condition called uremia. Uremia is a serious condition that can cause a wide range of symptoms, such as nausea, vomiting, confusion, and even coma. It's important to detect and treat kidney disease early to prevent these symptoms.

Chronic kidney disease (CKD) is a gradual loss of kidney function over time, it can happen over months to years and can lead to kidney failure. The most common causes of CKD include diabetes, hypertension and glomerulonephritis. Symptoms of CKD include fatigue, difficulty concentrating, difficulty sleeping, and frequent urination.

Kidney disease can also lead to other health problems, such as anemia, bone disease, and cardiovascular disease. That's why early detection and treatment is critical to prevent progression of the disease and the development of these complications.

The kidneys are complex organs and the symptoms of kidney disease are often subtle, so it is important to work with a healthcare professional to detect and manage kidney disease. This includes regular check-ups and blood tests to monitor kidney function and detect any problems early. Treatment may include medications, lifestyle changes, and in advanced cases, dialysis or kidney transplantation.

In conclusion, the kidneys play a vital role in maintaining overall health by filtering waste products from the blood, regulating electrolyte balance and producing hormones that are important for maintaining homeostasis in the body. However, when the kidneys are not functioning properly, waste products can build up in the blood, leading to serious health problems such as chronic kidney disease. It is important to detect and treat kidney disease early to prevent progression of the disease and the development of complications.

2

Epidemiology and causes of kidney disease

Kidney disease, also known as chronic kidney disease (CKD), is a significant public health issue affecting millions of people worldwide. Epidemiology is the study of the frequency and distribution of disease in a population, and understanding the epidemiology of kidney disease can help in developing strategies for preventing and managing the disease.

According to the National Kidney Foundation, 26 million adults in the United States have CKD, and millions more are at risk for developing the disease. The incidence of kidney disease varies by demographic and geographic factors. Age is a major risk factor for kidney disease, with the incidence increasing with age. Additionally, certain racial and ethnic groups are at higher risk for kidney disease, including African Americans, Hispanic Americans, American Indians, and Pacific Islanders.

Diabetes is one of the most common causes of kidney disease, with the Centers for Disease Control and Prevention (CDC) reporting that diabetes is responsible for approximately 44% of new cases of kidney failure. People with diabetes have high blood sugar levels, which can damage the blood vessels in the kidneys over time. This damage can cause the kidneys to work less effectively, resulting in the buildup of waste products in the bloodstream.

Hypertension, or high blood pressure, is another leading cause of kidney disease and is responsible for approximately 25% of new cases of kidney failure. High blood pressure can damage the blood vessels in the kidneys, causing them to work less effectively. People with hypertension also have an increased risk of developing diabetic kidney disease.

Other common causes of kidney disease include genetic conditions, such as polycystic kidney disease and inherited kidney disease, as well as autoimmune disorders, such as lupus and IgA nephropathy. These conditions can cause inflammation and damage to the kidneys, leading to dysfunction.

Certain medications can also cause kidney damage, such as non-steroidal anti-inflammatory drugs (NSAIDs) and certain antibiotics. Long-term use of these medications can cause nephrotoxicity, or damage to the kidneys. Toxins and pollution can also damage the kidneys over time, leading to disease.

Other causes include chronic kidney infections, physical injuries in the kidneys, and long-term use of nephrotoxic drugs. Individuals with a history of kidney diseases in their families are also at a higher risk of developing the disease themselves.

In addition to these risk factors, lifestyle factors such as smoking, lack of physical activity, and poor diet can also increase the risk of developing kidney disease. These factors can contribute to the development of diabetes and hypertension, as well as cause other health problems such as obesity, which can increase the risk of kidney disease.

It is important to note that early detection and management of kidney disease can prevent or delay the need for dialysis or transplantation. Regular check-ups and screenings with a healthcare professional can help to detect kidney disease early and prevent the progression of the disease.

In conclusion, kidney disease, also known as chronic kidney disease (CKD), is a significant public health issue that affects millions of people worldwide. The incidence of the disease varies by demographic and geographic factors, with older individuals and certain racial and ethnic groups at a higher risk. The most common causes of kidney disease are diabetes and hypertension, but other causes include genetic conditions, autoimmune disorders, and certain medications. Lifestyle factors such as poor diet, lack of physical activity and smoking also contribute to the development of the disease. Early detection and management of the disease can prevent or delay the need for dialysis or transplantation.

CHAPTER 2

Understanding Chronic Kidney Disease

Chronic kidney disease (CKD) is a condition in which the kidneys gradually lose function over time. The kidneys are two bean-shaped organs located on either side of the spine that filter waste and excess fluids from the bloodstream. In early stages of CKD, there may be few or no symptoms. However, as the disease progresses, the kidneys may not be able to properly filter waste, which can lead to a build-up of toxins in the body. This can cause a variety of health problems, including anemia, bone disease, and heart disease.

There are several causes of CKD, including diabetes, hypertension (high blood pressure), and genetic disorders. Diabetes and hypertension are the two most common causes of CKD, accounting for around two-thirds of cases. When diabetes and hypertension are well-controlled, the progression of CKD can often be slowed or even halted.

Symptoms of CKD include fatigue, weakness, difficulty concentrating, decreased appetite, nausea, and swelling in the legs and ankles. In advanced stages of CKD, symptoms may include difficulty urinating, persistent itching, and blood in the urine. As the disease progresses, the kidneys may not be able to produce enough erythropoietin (a hormone that helps the body produce red blood cells), leading to anemia. This can cause fatigue, weakness, and shortness of breath.

Diagnosis of CKD typically begins with a physical examination, including a review of the patient's medical history and a test of their urine for protein (albumin) and blood. Blood tests will be done to measure the creatinine and estimated glomerular filtration rate (eGFR) which gives an indication of how well the kidneys are functioning. For advanced stages or suspected causes, further tests such as Ultrasound, CT scan, MRI or kidney biopsy may be done.

Treatment for CKD typically involves controlling the underlying condition that is causing the disease. In the case of diabetes or hypertension, this may involve taking medication to lower blood sugar or blood pressure. Additionally, a diet low in salt, protein, and potassium may be recommended to slow the progression of the disease. When the disease has progressed to an advanced stage and the kidneys can no longer function properly, dialysis or kidney transplantation may be necessary.

In addition to medical treatment, there are several things that patients with CKD can do to manage their condition. This include regular exercise, maintaining a healthy weight, and eating a healthy diet that is low in salt, potassium, and protein. Avoiding smoking and limiting alcohol consumption can also help to slow the progression of the disease.

It is important to monitor the condition closely, and people with CKD should schedule regular check-ups with a healthcare provider. If you are at high risk of developing CKD, such as people with diabetes or hypertension, or those with a family history of kidney disease, it's important to have regular kidney function test done. Early detection and treatment can help to slow the progression of the disease, reduce the risk of complications, and improve quality of life.

In summary, Chronic Kidney Disease (CKD) is a serious medical condition in which the kidneys gradually lose function over time. It is commonly caused by diabetes and hypertension and can lead to a variety of health problems. Symptoms may not be present in the early stages, but as the disease progresses, it can lead to fatigue, weakness, and difficulty concentrating. A diagnosis is made by a physical examination and blood and urine tests. Treatment options include controlling the underlying condition, medications, diet, and in advanced stages, dialysis or kidney transplantation. With early detection, appropriate treatment and management, the progression of the disease can be slowed and the risk of complications can be reduced. It is crucial for individuals who are at high risk of developing CKD to have regular kidney function tests and schedule regular check-ups with a healthcare provider to ensure early detection and appropriate management of the disease. Furthermore, lifestyle changes such as maintaining a healthy diet, regular exercise and avoiding smoking and limiting alcohol consumption can also play a critical role in slowing the progression of the disease and improving overall quality of life.

In addition to medical treatment, it's important for individuals with CKD to be mindful of emotional and psychological well-being. Chronic illness can have a significant emotional and psychological impact and It may be beneficial to seek support from a counselor, therapist or a support group. Coping with the physical and emotional challenges of CKD can be challenging, but with the help of healthcare professionals and emotional support, individuals with CKD can work to manage their condition and improve their quality of life.

In conclusion, Chronic Kidney Disease (CKD) is a serious condition that affects the kidneys over time and can lead to a variety of health problems if not properly managed. Early detection, management and monitoring are crucial to slowing the progression of the disease and reducing the risk of complications. Lifestyle changes, regular check-ups and emotional support can play a critical role in managing the condition and improving the overall quality of life for individuals with CKD.

4

Stages of chronic kidney disease

hronic kidney disease (CKD) is a progressive condition that affects the kidneys over time. It is typically characterized by a gradual decline in kidney function, which can lead to a variety of health problems if not properly managed. CKD is typically classified into five stages, with stage 1 being the earliest stage and stage 5 being the most advanced.

Stage 1: Normal or slightly decreased kidney function with an estimated glomerular filtration rate (eGFR) of 90 or above. At this stage, there are usually no symptoms and the individual may not even know they have CKD.

Stage 2: Mildly decreased kidney function with an eGFR between 60 and 89. At this stage, there are still no symptoms and the individual may not know they have CKD. However, there may be slight abnormalities in the urine or blood tests, which can indicate the presence of the disease.

Stage 3: Moderately decreased kidney function with an eGFR between 30 and 59. At this stage, the individual may begin to experience symptoms such as fatigue, weakness, and difficulty concentrating. There may also be anemia, which can cause fatigue and shortness of breath. The individual may also experience swelling in the legs and ankles.

Stage 4: Severely decreased kidney function with an eGFR between 15 and 29. At this stage, the individual may experience symptoms such as difficulty urinating, persistent itching, and blood in the urine. They may also experience a decline in their overall health and an increased risk of complications such as cardiovascular disease. Dialysis may be needed in this stage

Stage 5: Kidney failure (an eGFR of less than 15) At this stage, the kidneys are no longer able to function properly and the individual will require dialysis or a kidney transplant to survive. Symptoms may include nausea, vomiting, fatigue, and loss of appetite. The individual may also be at risk of developing other complications such as infections, blood clots, and metabolic disorders.

It is important to note that the stages of CKD are not always linear and some individuals may progress rapidly while others may progress more slowly. Additionally, CKD is not always caused by one condition and multiple risk factors, such as diabetes and hypertension, may also lead to the disease.

Early detection and management of CKD is crucial to slowing the progression of the disease and reducing the risk of complications. This may involve controlling the underlying condition that is causing the disease, such as diabetes or hypertension, as well as making lifestyle changes such as main- taining a healthy diet, exercise and taking medications as prescribed. Regular monitoring by a healthcare provider is essential for managing the disease and preventing complications.

In summary, Chronic Kidney Disease (CKD) is a progressive condition that affects the kidneys over time, it is typically classified into five stages based on the estimated glomerular filtration rate (eGFR) which serves as an indicator of the level of kidney function. The stage ranges from stage 1 to 5 with 1 being the earliest and 5 the most advanced. At each stage the symptoms and complications are different. It is essential to have early detection, management and monitoring by a healthcare provider to slow the progression of the disease and reduce the risk of complications.

5

Symptoms and diagnosis

Symptoms Of CKD

Chronic kidney disease (CKD) is a condition in which the kidneys gradually lose function over time. The kidneys are two bean-shaped organs located on either side of the spine that filter waste and excess fluids from the bloodstream. In the early stages of CKD, there may be few or no symptoms. However, as the disease progresses, the kidneys may not be able to properly filter waste, which can lead to a build-up of toxins in the body. This can cause a variety of health problems, including anemia, bone disease, and heart disease. It is important to be aware of the symptoms of CKD to detect the disease early and to receive proper treatment.

- Fatigue and weakness: This can be caused by anemia, which occurs when the kidneys are not able to produce enough erythropoietin (a hormone that helps the body produce red blood cells). Fatigue and weakness can also be caused by the build-up of toxins in the body, which can affect overall energy levels.

- Difficulty concentrating: The build-up of toxins in the body can affect cognitive function and make it difficult to focus.

- Decreased appetite and nausea: As the kidneys lose function, they may not be able to remove waste from the bloodstream effectively, leading to nausea and decreased appetite.

- Swelling in the legs and ankles: When the kidneys are not functioning properly, fluids can build up in the body, leading to swelling in the legs and ankles.

- Difficulty urinating: As the disease progresses, the kidneys may not be able to produce enough urine, leading to difficulty urinating. This can include frequent urination, difficulty starting to urinate, and a weak urine stream.

- Persistent itching: The build-up of toxins in the body can cause itching, particularly on the legs and arms.

- Blood in the urine: As the disease progresses, the kidneys may not be able to filter waste effectively, leading to blood in the urine. This is also known as hematuria.

- Shortness of breath: Anemia caused by CKD can lead to shortness of breath.

- Chest pain and muscle cramps: As kidneys lose function, it can cause accumulation of minerals in the blood and cause chest pain or muscle cramps.

- Hypertension: High blood pressure is common in people with CKD, and uncontrolled hypertension can further damage the kidneys.

- Dry, itchy skin: As the kidneys lose function, they may not be able to remove waste and excess fluids from the bloodstream effectively, leading to dry, itchy skin.

- Bone pain: CKD can lead to bone disease, which can cause pain and weakness in the bones.

- Headaches: The build-up of toxins in the body can cause headaches and other symptoms of toxicity.

- Insomnia: Difficulty sleeping may also occur due to anemia, build-up of toxins, and other symptoms of CKD.

- Depression: Chronic illness can have an emotional and psychological impact, and individuals with CKD may be at an increased risk of depression.

It's important to note that the symptoms of CKD may vary from person to person and may not always be specific to the disease. For example, fatigue, weakness, and difficulty concentrating can be caused by a variety of other conditions as well. Additionally, some individuals may experience symptoms at an earlier stage of the disease than others. Therefore, it is important to have regular check-ups with a healthcare provider and to discuss any concerns or symptoms with them.

In conclusion, Chronic Kidney Disease (CKD) is a condition that causes gradual loss of kidney function over time and can lead to a variety of health problems if not properly managed. The symptoms may vary from person to person and may not always be specific to the disease. The early stages of CKD may cause few or no symptoms, but as the disease progresses, symptoms such as fatigue, weakness, difficulty concentrating, decreased appetite, nausea, swelling in the legs and ankles, difficulty urinating, persistent itching, blood in the urine, shortness of breath, chest pain, muscle cramps, hypertension, dry itchy skin, bone pain, headaches, insomnia and depression may appear. It is important to be aware of the symptoms of CKD and to have regular check-ups with a healthcare provider to detect the disease early and to receive proper treatment.

6

Diagnosis of CKD

The diagnosis of Chronic Kidney Disease (CKD) typically begins with a physical examination, including a review of the patient's medical history, symptoms, and a physical examination. Medical history can provide important information about possible risk factors for CKD, such as hypertension, diabetes, and a family history of kidney disease.

1. Urine tests:

A urine test will be done to look for protein (albumin) in the urine. Protein in the urine is called proteinuria, and it can be an early sign of CKD. A urine test will also be done to check the levels of red blood cells in the urine, which can indicate kidney damage.

2. Blood tests:

Blood tests will be done to measure the creatinine and estimated glomerular filtration rate (eGFR). Creatinine is a waste product produced by muscle metabolism and filtered by the kidneys, so if the kidneys are not working properly, creatinine levels in the blood will be higher. The eGFR uses the creatinine level to estimate how well the kidneys are working. A low eGFR means that the kidneys are not functioning properly. The National Kidney Foundation (NKF) recommends that adults over age 60 and adults with risk factors for kidney disease be screened for CKD every 3 years with the creatinine test.

3. Imaging tests:

In addition to physical examination and blood and urine tests, imaging tests may be done to check the size and shape of the kidneys and to look for any abnormalities. These tests can include ultrasound, CT scan, MRI, and angiography. An ultrasound uses sound waves to create a picture of the kidneys, which can show the size and shape of the organs and can help identify any abnormalities or blockages. CT scans and MRI's can provide detailed images of the kidneys, which can help to identify abnormalities or blockages. Angiography is a test that uses X-rays and a special dye to create detailed images of the blood vessels in the kidneys.

4. Kidney biopsy:

In cases where the cause of CKD is not clear, a kidney biopsy may be done. During a kidney biopsy, a small sample of tissue is taken from the kidney and examined under a microscope. This can help to determine the cause of CKD and to guide treatment.

It's important to note that diagnosis of CKD can be complex, and it is important to work closely with your healthcare provider to develop an appropriate treatment plan based on the specific cause of your condition. If you have symptoms or are at risk for CKD, it is important to schedule regular check-ups with a healthcare provider to monitor your kidney function and to detect any changes early.

In conclusion, the diagnosis of chronic kidney disease (CKD) typically involves a physical examination, review of medical history, and a series of tests that include urine and blood tests, imaging tests and kidney biopsy. Urine test helps to detect protein in the urine and red blood cells, which can be signs of CKD. Blood tests such as creatinine and estimated glomerular filtration rate (eGFR) can indicate the level of kidney function. Imaging tests such as ultrasound, CT scan, MRI and Angiography can be done to get an idea about the size and shape of the kidneys and to look for abnormalities or blockages. While kidney biopsy is done in cases where cause of CKD is not clear. It is crucial for individuals who are at high risk of developing CKD, to have regular check-ups with a healthcare provider and to work closely with the healthcare provider to develop an appropriate treatment plan for the specific cause of their condition.

7

CHAPTER 3

Conventional Treatment for Chronic Kidney Disease

Chronic kidney disease (CKD) is a progressive condition in which the kidneys lose their ability to function properly over time. Conventional treatment for CKD typically includes a combination of lifestyle changes, medication, and, in advanced cases, dialysis or kidney transplant.

Lifestyle changes that are recommended for people with CKD include maintaining a healthy diet that is low in salt, potassium, and phosphorus, and quitting smoking. A dietitian can help create a customized meal plan that is tailored to a patient's specific needs.

Medications are used to control symptoms and slow the progression of CKD. These include angiotensin-converting enzyme (ACE) inhibitors and angiotensin receptor blockers (ARBs), which help to lower blood pressure and reduce the workload on the kidneys. Additionally, diuretics, which remove excess fluid from the body, and phosphate binders, which help to lower phosphorus levels, are also commonly prescribed.

As CKD progresses, the kidneys lose more and more of their ability to filter waste products from the blood. When the kidneys are no longer able to function on their own, dialysis is used to take over the job of filtering the blood. Dialysis is typically performed either at a dialysis center or at home, and is typically done three times a week for several hours at a time.

When CKD reaches the end-stage, a kidney transplant may be recommended. A kidney transplant involves surgically removing the diseased kidneys and replacing them with a healthy kidney from a donor. The donated kidney can come from a living donor or from a deceased donor. After a successful transplant, the patient will no longer need dialysis, and most will have a better quality of life with improved kidney function.

It's important to note that conventional treatment for CKD is directed towards slowing the progression of the disease and managing symptoms, but it does not cure the underlying problem. It's essential to attend regularly check-ups with your nephrologist, follow your medication regimen and take other necessary precautions to prevent complications. Additionally, early detection and management of CKD can slow its progression and prevent or delay the need for dialysis or transplant.

In summary, conventional treatment for CKD includes a combination of lifestyle changes, medication, dialysis and kidney transplant, but the specific treatment plan will vary depending on the individual case, stage and overall health condition of the patient. Close monitoring of the patient's condition is a vital part of the treatment plan, and early detection and management can significantly improve outcomes.

8

Understanding The Risk factors For CKD

hronic kidney disease (CKD) is a condition in which the kidneys gradually lose function over time. There are several risk factors that can increase a person's risk of developing CKD. Understanding these risk factors can help individuals take steps to reduce their risk and to detect the disease early.

Diabetes: Diabetes is one of the most common causes of CKD. High blood sugar levels can damage the blood vessels in the kidneys, leading to a gradual loss of function. People with diabetes should have regular check-ups with a healthcare provider and have their kidney function tested at least once a year.

Hypertension (high blood pressure): High blood pressure can damage the blood vessels in the kidneys, leading to a gradual loss of function. People with hypertension should have regular check-ups with a healthcare provider and have their kidney function tested at least once a year.

Family history: A family history of kidney disease can increase a person's risk of developing CKD. If a person has a family history of kidney disease, they should have regular check-ups with a healthcare provider and have their kidney function tested at least once a year.

Age: As people get older, the risk of developing CKD increases. The National Kidney Foundation (NKF) recommends that adults over age 60 and adults with risk factors for kidney disease be screened for CKD every 3 years.

Ethnicity: Some ethnic groups, such as African Americans, Hispanics, and American Indians, are at an increased risk of developing CKD.

Obesity: Being overweight or obese can increase the risk of CKD. Obesity can cause diabetes, hypertension and other conditions that increase the risk of CKD.

Smoking: Smoking can increase the risk of CKD by damaging the blood vessels in the kidneys. It can also increase the risk of hypertension, diabetes, and other conditions that can lead to CKD.

Cardiovascular disease: Having conditions such as heart disease, coronary artery disease, and peripheral artery disease can increase the risk of CKD. These conditions can damage the blood vessels in the kidneys and lead to a gradual loss of function.

Certain medications: Some medications, such as non-steroidal anti-inflammatory drugs (NSAIDs) and some antibiotics, can damage the kidneys. Long-term use of these medications should be done with caution, and under the supervision of healthcare provider.

Environmental toxins: Exposure to certain environmental toxins, such as lead and cadmium, can increase the risk of CKD.

Chronic infections: Chronic infections such as HIV and Hepatitis B and C can increase the risk of CKD by damaging the kidneys.

Renal artery stenosis: This is a condition in which the renal artery that brings blood to the kidneys is narrowed. This can cause hypertension and lead to kidney damage.

It's important to note that having one or more of these risk factors does not guarantee that a person will develop CKD. However, individuals who have one or more risk factors should be aware of their risk and take steps to reduce their risk. This includes maintaining a healthy lifestyle, controlling any underlying medical conditions, and having regular check-ups with a healthcare provider.

In conclusion, Chronic Kidney Disease (CKD) is a condition in which the kidneys gradually lose function over time. There are several risk factors that can increase a person's risk of developing CKD, including diabetes, hypertension, family history, age, ethnicity, obesity, smoking, cardiovascular disease, certain medications, environmental toxins, chronic infections and Renal artery stenosis. It's important for individuals who have one or more risk factors to be aware of their risk and to take steps to reduce their risk by maintaining a healthy lifestyle, controlling any underlying medical conditions, and having regular check-ups with a healthcare provider.

9

Medication For Hypertension

Hypertension, or high blood pressure, is a common condition that occurs when the force of blood against the walls of the arteries is too high. This can lead to serious health problems, including heart disease, stroke, and kidney failure, if left untreated. Medications used to control hypertension, or high blood pressure, include diuretics, beta blockers, ACE inhibitors, calcium channel blockers, and angiotensin receptor blockers.

Diuretics, also known as "water pills," work by increasing the amount of salt and water that the kidneys remove from the bloodstream. This leads to an increase in urine output, which in turn reduces the volume of blood in the circulatory system. This reduces the pressure on the blood vessels, lowering blood pressure. Thiazide diuretics are the most common type of diuretics prescribed for hypertension. They're particularly effective in people with hypertension and are often used as the first line of treatment. Loop diuretics are used in more severe cases or when thiazides are not effective. They increase the amount of salt and water excreted in the urine even more effectively than thiazides.

Beta blockers slow the heart rate and reduce the force of the heart's contractions. This reduces the workload on the heart, allowing blood to flow more easily through the circulatory system. This reduces the pressure on the blood vessels, lowering blood pressure. Beta blockers are most commonly used to treat hypertension and other heart conditions, such as angina and heart failure. Some examples of beta blockers used to treat hypertension include metoprolol, atenolol, and propranolol.

ACE inhibitors and angiotensin receptor blockers both work by blocking the action of a substance in the body called angiotensin II, which causes blood vessels to constrict and raises blood pressure. ACE inhibitors, such as lisinopril, captopril, and ramipril, are a widely used class of hypertension medications that are particularly effective in people with diabetes, kidney disease, and heart failure. Angiotensin receptor blockers (ARBs) such as losartan, valsartan, and irbesartan, work by preventing angiotensin II from binding to its receptors on the blood vessels, which causes the blood vessels to relax and lowers blood pressure.

Calcium channel blockers slow the movement of calcium into the muscle cells of the heart and blood vessels, which causes the blood vessels to relax and lowers blood pressure. Calcium channel blockers are often used to treat hypertension, angina, and certain heart rhythm disorders. Some examples of calcium channel blockers used to treat hypertension include amlodipine, diltiazem, and verapamil.

It's also important to note that, hypertension medication usually need to be taken long-term and that doctors may need to try different combinations or dosages of medications before finding the most effective treatment plan for a person. Lifestyle changes such as eating a healthy diet, getting regular exercise, and maintaining a healthy weight are also essential in the management of hypertension, and may allow some people to avoid medication or reduce the dosage required to control their blood pressure.

However, it's important to follow the treatment plan recommended by your healthcare provider and to not discontinue taking your medications without consulting a healthcare professional, as abruptly stopping hypertension medication can cause a rapid increase in blood pressure which could lead to a stroke or heart attack.

It's also important to regularly check your blood pressure and keep track of any changes. This will help your healthcare provider to adjust your treatment plan as needed.

Medication for lowering cholesterol

Cholesterol is a type of fat found in the blood that plays an important role in maintaining the health of the body. However, high levels of cholesterol can lead to a buildup of plaque in the arteries, which can increase the risk of heart disease and stroke. To lower cholesterol levels, there are several types of medications that can be prescribed by a healthcare provider.

One class of medications for lowering cholesterol is called statins. These drugs work by inhibiting the enzyme that is responsible for producing cholesterol in the liver. This leads to a decrease in the amount of LDL, or "bad" cholesterol, in the blood. Statins are considered to be the first-line therapy for high cholesterol and have been shown to be effective in reducing the risk of heart attack and stroke. Examples of statins include atorvastatin (Lipitor), simvastatin (Zocor), and rosuvastatin (Crestor).

Another class of medications that can be used to lower cholesterol is called bile acid sequestrants. These drugs work by binding to bile acids in the intestines and preventing them from being reabsorbed into the bloodstream. This leads to an increase in the amount of bile acids being removed from the body, which in turn leads to an increase in the production of LDL cholesterol in the liver. This class of drugs has been shown to be effective in reducing the levels of LDL cholesterol. Examples of bile acid sequestrants include cholestyramine (Questran) and colestipol (Colestid).

A third class of medications for lowering cholesterol are known as ezetimibe drugs, which works by inhibiting the absorption of cholesterol in the small intestine. ezetimibe is often used in combination with statins to help achieve optimal cholesterol levels. An example of ezetimibe is Zetia.

Niacin, also known as vitamin B3, is another medication that can be used to lower cholesterol levels. Niacin works by increasing the production of HDL, or "good" cholesterol, in the body. Niacin has been shown to be effective in reducing the levels of LDL cholesterol and increasing the levels of HDL cholesterol. However, the high doses required for cholesterol lowering can cause side effects such as flushing, itching, and nausea.

Finally, new class of drugs called PCSK9 inhibitors, like evolocumab (Repatha) and alirocumab (Praluent) can be prescribed to patients who are unable to achieve sufficient LDL cholesterol lowering with statins alone. These drugs are monoclonal antibodies and block the proprotein convertase subtilisin/kexin type 9 (PCSK9) protein which is responsible for LDL receptor degradation.

It is important to note that lifestyle changes such as a healthy diet, regular exercise, and weight management can also help lower cholesterol levels. Medications should be used in conjunction with these lifestyle changes for optimal results.

In conclusion, there are several types of medications that can be used to lower cholesterol levels. These include statins, bile acid sequestrants, ezetimibe, niacin and PCSK9 inhibitors. These medications can be effective in reducing the risk of heart disease and stroke. However, they should be used in conjunction with lifestyle changes such as a healthy diet, regular exercise, and weight management for optimal results. Always consult with a healthcare provider before starting any medication regimen.

Medications for slowing progression of CKD

Chronic kidney disease (CKD) is a gradual loss of kidney function over time, it can happen over months to years and can lead to kidney failure. Medications can play an important role in slowing the progression of kidney disease and managing the symptoms associated with CKD.

One of the most important medications for slowing the progression of kidney disease is ACE inhibitors or ARBs (angiotensin receptor blockers). These medications work by blocking the action of a hormone called angiotensin II, which causes blood vessels to constrict and raises blood pressure. By blocking this hormone, ACE inhibitors and ARBs can lower blood pressure and reduce the strain on the kidneys. They also have been shown to reduce the risk of kidney disease progression and cardiovascular disease in people with diabetes and hypertension.

Another important class of medications for slowing the progression of kidney disease are diuretics, also known as water pills. They increase the excretion of water and sodium in the urine and reduce blood volume which reduces the burden on the kidneys and also lowers blood pressure. Thiazide diuretics are commonly used to lower blood pressure and are often used in combination with ACE inhibitors or ARBs.

Another important class of drugs for slowing the progression of kidney disease is phosphate binder which bind the phosphorus in the diet and prevent it from being absorbed into the bloodstream. High levels of phosphorus can lead to bone disease and hardening of the arteries, which can accelerate kidney disease progression. Calcium-based binders are the most commonly used binders and they can also help correct low calcium levels that can occur in people with kidney disease.

Medications that lower cholesterol levels like statins are also important for slowing the progression of kidney disease. High cholesterol levels are a risk factor for cardiovascular disease and can accelerate kidney disease progression. Statins can lower the risk of cardiovascular disease and slow the progression of kidney disease by reducing the amount of cholesterol in the blood.

Anemia, a common complication of kidney disease, is caused by a lack of erythropoietin, a hormone produced by the kidneys that stimulates the production of red blood cells. People with CKD may develop anemia, which can cause fatigue, shortness of breath, and other symptoms. Erythropoiesis-stimulating agents (ESAs) can be used to treat anemia in people with kidney disease. These medications stimulate the production of red blood cells and can improve symptoms of anemia and reduce the need for blood transfusions. However, the use of ESAs should be carefully monitored, as high doses or overuse can increase the risk of blood clots, stroke, and death.

Lastly, pain management medications such as non-steroidal anti-inflammatory drugs (NSAIDs) can be used to control pain and inflammation in people with kidney disease. However, NSAIDs should be used with caution in people with kidney disease, as they can cause further damage to the kidneys and should be avoided in cases of advanced kidney disease.

It's important to note that every individual case of kidney disease is unique, so the treatment will vary. Not all medications may be appropriate for everyone and some may have side effects. It's crucial to consult a medical professional or a nephrologist (kidney specialist) to assess the condition and choose the most appropriate medications.

In addition to medication, lifestyle changes such as maintaining a healthy diet, regular physical activity, and avoiding smoking and excessive alcohol consumption can also help to slow the progression of kidney disease.

In conclusion, Medications play a crucial role in slowing the progression of kidney disease and managing the symptoms associated with it. Medications such as ACE inhibitors, ARBs, diuretics, phosphate binders, statins, erythropoiesis-stimulating agents, and pain management medications can be used to slow the progression of kidney disease, However, it is important to work closely with a healthcare professional to determine the best treatment plan, as individual cases of kidney disease vary

11

Dialysis And its Types

Dialysis

Dialysis is a medical treatment that is used to remove waste products and excess fluid from the blood when the kidneys are not able to function properly. The kidneys are responsible for filtering waste products and excess fluid from the blood, but when they are not able to do this effectively, it can lead to a buildup of these substances in the blood which can be dangerous. Dialysis helps to remove these substances and keep the blood clean, ensuring the proper functioning of other organs and the maintenance of overall health.

There are two main types of dialysis: hemodialysis and peritoneal dialysis. Hemodialysis is the most common type of dialysis, and it uses a machine to filter the blood. During hemodialysis, a patient's blood is removed from the body and passed through an artificial kidney (dialysis machine) that filters out the waste products, and then returned to the body. Hemodialysis is typically done in a hospital or dialysis center and is usually done three times a week for about four hours per treatment.

In Hemodialysis, a patient needs to have access to the bloodstream, this is achieved by surgically creating an access, either a fistula (joining an artery and a vein) or a graft (synthetic tube) that will be used to connect the patient's blood vessels to the dialysis machine. This allows blood to flow out of the body, into the dialysis machine, where it is filtered and cleaned, before being returned to the body. The artificial kidney, also called a dialysis membrane, is made of a semi-permeable material that allows waste products and excess fluids to pass through while retaining important molecules such as red blood cells.

Peritoneal dialysis is another type of dialysis that uses the patient's own peritoneal membrane, which lines the abdominal cavity, to filter the blood. This is done by filling the patient's abdominal cavity with a special solution called dialysis solution that absorbs waste products and excess fluids from the blood. A tube called a catheter is surgically implanted into the patient's abdomen to allow for the exchange of fluids. The used dialysis solution is then drained from the patient's body and replaced with fresh solution. Peritoneal dialysis can be done at home and does not require a machine. It is done daily for about 4-5 hours per treatment, and it can be performed during the day or overnight while sleeping.

During both types of dialysis, waste products that are removed from the blood include urea, creatinine, and potassium. Fluids that are removed include excess water and electrolytes like sodium. In addition, dialysis can also help to control blood pressure, and alleviate symptoms such as fatigue, edema, or anemia. Hemodialysis and Peritoneal dialysis are both effective treatments, however, each one has its own set of benefits and drawbacks. The choice between the two options will often depend on individual patient's lifestyle, medical condition, and personal preference.

Dialysis can be a life-saving treatment for those with kidney failure, however, it can also have its own set of complications. Hemodialysis can be associated with access site problems, bleeding, hypotension, and infections. Peritoneal dialysis can lead to infection or blockage of the catheter and long-term complications such as peritonitis and hernias. Additionally, both types of dialysis can cause physical discomfort, and emotional toll, it can be demanding on the patient's time and can be expensive.

Kidney transplantation is also an option for people with kidney failure, it is considered a more effective treatment than dialysis and can improve quality of life and longevity. However, it is not suitable for everyone and the availability of a suitable donor is limited.

In conclusion, Dialysis is a medical treatment that is used to remove waste products and excess fluid from the blood when the kidneys are not able to function properly. Hemodialysis and Peritoneal dialysis are the two main types of dialysis, and they are both effective treatment options. However, they also have their own set of complications and they are not suitable for everyone. A kidney transplantation is also an option, which is a more effective treatment than dialysis and can improve quality of life and longevity. It's important to work closely with a healthcare professional to determine the best treatment plan, as individual cases of kidney disease vary. It's crucial for people with kidney disease to be informed about all treatment options available for them, to make an informed decision about the best course of treatment for their condition.

12

Kidney Transplation

Kidney Transplation Process

Kidney transplantation is a surgical procedure that is used to treat end-stage renal disease, also known as kidney failure. The procedure involves replacing a person's diseased or damaged kidneys with a healthy donor kidney. The transplantation process can greatly improve a person's quality of life and longevity, as it eliminates the need for dialysis and allows the person to return to a more normal life.

The first step in the kidney transplantation process is to determine if the person is a candidate for a transplant. This includes a thorough evaluation to ensure that the person is in good enough health to undergo the surgery and that the person does not have any other medical conditions that would make the transplant a high-risk procedure. This evaluation includes blood tests, imaging studies, and consultations with various specialists, such as a transplant surgeon, a nephrologist, a cardiologist, and a psychologist.

Once it has been determined that a person is a suitable candidate for a transplant, the next step is to find a donor kidney. There are two types of donors, living donors, and deceased donors. Living donors are typically a close relative, such as a parent, sibling, or child, while deceased donors are individuals who have recently died and have agreed to donate their organs. In both cases, the donors' kidneys are evaluated to ensure that they are suitable for transplantation.

Once a suitable donor kidney is found, the next step is the actual transplant surgery. The surgery is typically done under general anesthesia and can take several hours to complete. The transplanted kidney is typically placed in the lower abdomen, and the blood vessels of the new kidney are connected to the person's own vessels. The person's own kidneys are not removed during the procedure, but they will not function.

After the surgery, the person will need to stay in the hospital for a few days to recover. Close monitoring will be done for several days to ensure the transplant kidney is functioning well and to detect any complications. Medications will be prescribed to help prevent rejection, which is the body's immune system's attempt to reject the new kidney.

After the transplant, the person will need to take immunosuppressant drugs to prevent the body from rejecting the new kidney. These drugs suppress the immune system, making it less likely to attack the new kidney. This medication will be taken for the rest of the person's life.

The recovery period after a transplant can vary, but typically it can take several weeks to several months to fully recover. It is important to have regular follow-up care with the transplant team to monitor the function of the new kidney, and to adjust the immunosuppressant dose as needed. The transplant team will also monitor for any signs of rejection or infection, which can occur at any time after the transplant.

In addition to monitoring the transplant kidney's function, it's important to also maintain a healthy lifestyle, including a healthy diet and regular physical activity, and to attend all scheduled clinic visits. It's important to be aware of the signs of rejection, such as fever, nausea, vomiting, lower back pain, and changes in urine output, and to report them promptly to the transplant team.

The success rate for kidney transplantation is quite high, with more than 80% of transplants still functioning well after one year. After five years, the success rate drops to about 70%, and after ten years, it is around 60%. However, it's important to note that a transplanted kidney can still fail, and if this happens, the person will need to return to dialysis or undergo another transplant.

In conclusion, kidney transplantation is a surgical procedure that is used to treat end-stage renal disease, or kidney failure. It involves replacing a person's diseased or damaged kidneys with a healthy donor kidney, which can greatly improve a person's quality of life and longevity. The transplantation process includes a thorough evaluation to ensure the person is a suitable candidate, finding a suitable donor, and the actual transplant surgery. After the transplant, the person will need to take immunosuppressant drugs to prevent rejection and to monitor the new kidney's function. It's important to have regular follow-up care, maintain a healthy lifestyle, and attend all scheduled clinic visits. Kidney transplantation has high success rates, but it is important to be aware that a transplanted kidney can still fail and the person may need to return to dialysis or undergo another transplant.

13

Evaluation Process For Kidney Transplant

Evaluation Process

The evaluation process for kidney transplantation is an important step to ensure that the person is a suitable candidate for the procedure. The evaluation process typically includes a thorough medical evaluation, a psychological evaluation, and a financial evaluation.

The medical evaluation includes a variety of tests and exams to determine the person's overall health, including blood tests, imaging studies, and consultations with various specialists such as a transplant surgeon, a nephrologist, a cardiologist, and an infectious disease specialist. The purpose of these tests is to ensure that the person is healthy enough to undergo the transplant surgery and to rule out any medical conditions that would make the transplant a high-risk procedure. Additionally, the medical evaluation will also assess the patient's other existing medical conditions and the effects of them on a potential transplant.

The psychological evaluation is also an important part of the evaluation process, as it assesses the person's emotional and mental well-being, as well as their support system. The transplant process can be a long and challenging one, both physically and emotionally, and it's important to have a support system in place. Additionally, psychological evaluation will help to identify any emotional issues or psychological disorders that might complicate the recovery process after the transplant.

The financial evaluation is also important, as it assesses the person's ability to afford the transplant and the necessary post-transplant care. The cost of a kidney transplant and the care required afterwards can be significant, and it's important to have a plan in place to cover these costs. It is important to have insurance that covers transplantation, however, not all insurance covers all the costs, and there are other costs that should be taken into account, such as transportation and medication.

Once a person is determined to be a suitable candidate for transplantation, the next step is to find a suitable donor kidney. There are two types of donors, living donors, and deceased donors. Living donors are typically a close relative such as a parent , sibling, or child, while deceased donors are individuals who have recently died and have agreed to donate their organs. In both cases, the donors' kidneys are evaluated to ensure that they are suitable for transplantation.

After the transplant, it is essential to have close monitoring, and regular follow-up care with the transplant team to ensure the transplant kidney is functioning well and to detect any complications. Post-transplant care includes immunosuppressant drugs to prevent rejection, which is the body's immune system's attempt to reject the new kidney. These drugs suppress the immune system, making it less likely to attack the new kidney. This medication will be taken for the rest of the person's life.

The transplant team will also closely monitor for any signs of rejection or infection, which can occur at any time after the transplant. It's important for the patient to be aware of the signs of rejection, such as fever, nausea, vomiting, lower back pain, and changes in urine output, and to report them promptly to the transplant team.

Regular follow-up visits, blood tests, and imaging studies will also be scheduled to monitor the transplant kidney's function and to detect any potential complications, such as rejection, infection, or damage to the new kidney. The transplant team will also monitor the patient's overall health and make any necessary adjustments to the treatment plan, such as adjusting the dose of immunosuppressant drugs.

In addition to the medical care, it is important to maintain a healthy lifestyle, including a healthy diet and regular physical activity, and to attend all scheduled clinic visits. Adhering to a strict medication regimen, avoiding smoking, excessive alcohol consumption and staying away from immunosuppressant drugs that can interact with the prescribed drugs, also is crucial.

In conclusion, the evaluation process for kidney transplantation is an important step to ensure that the person is a suitable candidate for the procedure. The evaluation process typically includes a thorough medical evaluation, a psychological evaluation, and a financial evaluation. These evaluations aim to ensure the person's overall health, emotional and mental well-being, and the availability of support system and resources to cover the costs of the transplant.

14

Chapter 4

Lifestyle and Alternative Solutions for Managing Chronic Kidney Disease

Maintaining a healthy diet is an important aspect of managing chronic kidney disease and preventing its progression. The kidneys play a vital role in maintaining the balance of fluids and minerals in the body and filtering waste products from the blood. However, when the kidneys are not functioning properly, it can lead to an accumulation of waste products in the blood, which can be harmful to the body. A healthy diet can help to support kidney function and promote overall health.

The National Kidney Foundation (NKF) recommends a kidney-friendly diet for people with chronic kidney disease. This diet focuses on controlling the intake of certain nutrients that can be harmful to the kidneys when they are not functioning properly.

Protein: The NKF recommends that people with chronic kidney disease limit their intake of protein. High protein intake can put a strain on the kidneys and can accelerate the progression of kidney disease. The NKF recommends that people with chronic kidney disease should consume 0.6 to 0.8 grams of protein per kilogram of body weight per day. This is equivalent to about 45 to 60 grams of protein per day for a 150-pound person.

Phosphorus: Phosphorus is a mineral that is found in many foods, and it is important for the proper functioning of the body. However, when the kidneys are not functioning properly, too much phosphorus can accumulate in the blood and cause problems. The NKF recommends that people with chronic kidney disease limit their intake of phosphorus to 800 to 1000 mg per day.

Potassium: Potassium is an essential mineral that is important for the proper functioning of the heart and muscles. However, when the kidneys are not functioning properly, too much potassium can accumulate in the blood and cause problems. The NKF recommends that people with chronic kidney disease limit their intake of potassium to 2000 to 2500 mg per day.

Fluid: The NKF also recommends that people with chronic kidney disease should limit their intake of fluid. This is because when the kidneys are not functioning properly, they may not be able to remove excess fluid from the body, which can cause swelling and high blood pressure. The NKF recommends that people with chronic kidney disease should limit their intake of fluid to about 32 to 48 ounces per day.

The NKF also recommends that people with chronic kidney disease should consume a diet that is low in saturated fat, cholesterol, and added sugars. A diet that is high in fruits, vegetables, and whole grains is also recommended.

It's important to note that dietary needs can vary depending on the stage of kidney disease and other existing medical conditions. It's essential to work closely with a registered dietitian or nephrologist to develop a personalized diet plan that is right for you.

In conclusion, maintaining a healthy diet is an important aspect of managing chronic kidney disease and preventing its progression. The National Kidney Foundation (NKF) recommends a kidney-friendly diet for people with chronic kidney disease, which focuses on controlling the intake of certain nutrients that can be harmful to the kidneys when they are not functioning properly. This includes limiting protein, phosphorus, potassium and fluids intake. It is also recommended to consume a diet that is low in saturated fat, cholesterol, and added sugars, and high in fruits, vegetables, and whole grains. It's important to note that dietary needs can vary depending on the stage of kidney disease and other existing medical conditions, which is why it's essential to work closely with a registered dietitian or nephrologist to develop a personalized diet plan that is right for you. It's also important to follow the recommended dietary guidelines in order to achieve optimal health and prevent further deterioration of kidney function.

15

The Importance of Exercise in Managing Chronic Kidney Disease (CKD)

Regular exercise is an important aspect of managing chronic kidney disease (CKD) and can help to improve overall health and quality of life. Exercise has been shown to have a number of benefits for people with CKD, including:

1. Improving cardiovascular health: Exercise can help to improve cardiovascular health by lowering blood pressure and cholesterol levels, which can help to reduce the risk of heart disease. This is particularly important for people with CKD, as they are at a higher risk of developing heart disease due to the accumulation of waste products in the blood.

2. Improving muscle strength and endurance: Exercise can help to improve muscle strength and endurance, which can help to improve overall physical function. This is particularly important for people with CKD, as they may experience muscle weakness and fatigue due to the accumulation of waste products in the blood.

3. Improving bone health: Exercise can help to improve bone health by increasing bone density and reducing the risk of osteoporosis. This is

particularly important for people with CKD, as they are at a higher risk of developing osteoporosis due to the accumulation of waste products in the blood.

4. Improving mental health: Exercise has been shown to have a positive impact on mental health, reducing symptoms of depression and anxiety. This is particularly important for people with CKD, as they may experience emotional distress due to their condition.

5. Improving quality of life: Exercise can help to improve overall quality of life by reducing symptoms of fatigue and improving physical function. This can help people with CKD to maintain their independence and continue to participate in activities they enjoy.

It's important to note that exercise should be tailored to the individual's abilities and should be done under the guidance of a healthcare professional. The exercise program should be designed to include both aerobic and resistance exercises, and should be adjusted as the patient's condition changes over time.

Aerobic exercises such as brisk walking, cycling, swimming, and dancing are good for cardiovascular health and endurance. Resistance exercises such as weightlifting or resistance band training are good for building muscle strength. Flexibility exercises such as yoga and stretching are also important to maintain range of motion, and balance exercises to prevent falls.

It's also important to note that people with CKD should avoid strenuous activities that could cause injury or strain on the kidneys, like contact sports, long-distance running or endurance events. Also, patients with advanced stages of CKD may need to avoid exercises that put extra pressure on the kidneys such as weightlifting or resistance training, and may need to focus on low-impact activities like walking or swimming.

In conclusion, regular exercise is an important aspect of managing chronic kidney disease (CKD) and can help to improve overall health and quality of life. Exercise can help to improve cardiovascular health, muscle strength and endurance, bone health, mental health and quality of life. It's important to tailor exercise to the individual's abilities and to do it under the guidance of a healthcare professional. A well-rounded exercise program should include both aerobic and resistance exercises, as well as flexibility and balance exercises. It's also important to avoid strenuous activities that could cause injury or strain on the kidneys and also adjust the exercise program as the patient's condition changes over time.

16

Herbs for Kidney Health

Herbs have been used for centuries to promote overall health and well-being, and this includes the health of the kidneys. The kidneys are an essential part of the body's filtration system and are responsible for removing waste products and excess fluids from the blood. They also play a crucial role in regulating blood pressure, electrolyte balance, and the production of hormones that control red blood cell production and promote bone health. When it comes to kidney health, there are several herbs that have been found to be beneficial.

One of the most commonly used herbs for kidney health is dandelion. Dandelion is a diuretic, which means it helps to increase urine output and flush out toxins and excess fluids from the body. It is also rich in antioxidants and has anti-inflammatory properties, which can help to protect the kidneys from damage caused by free radicals. Dandelion can be taken in the form of supplements, teas or even used in cooking.

Another popular herb for kidney health is cranberry. Cranberry is known for its ability to prevent urinary tract infections, but it also has properties that can help to protect the kidneys. Cranberry contains compounds called proanthocyanidins, which have been shown to inhibit the formation of kidney stones. It also has anti-inflammatory properties that can help to reduce inflammation in the kidneys, which can help to protect them from damage. Cranberry supplements, juice or even dried cranberries can be consumed to benefit the kidneys.

Another herb that is commonly used for kidney health is cornsilk. Cornsilk is a diuretic and has been used for centuries to help with urinary tract problems. It is rich in flavonoids and minerals, which can help to protect the kidneys from damage. Cornsilk is also high in potassium, which can help to regulate blood pressure and prevent hypertension, which is a leading cause of kidney disease. Cornsilk can be consumed in the form of tea or supplements.

Another herb that is known for its kidney-protective properties is parsley. Parsley is a natural diuretic, which can help to flush out toxins and excess fluids from the body. It is also rich in antioxidants and has anti-inflammatory properties, which can help to protect the kidneys from damage. Parsley can be consumed in the form of supplements, teas or can be used to garnish dishes.

Another herb that is beneficial for kidney health is juniper berries. Juniper berries have been used for centuries to help with urinary tract problems and kidney stones. They are known for their diuretic properties and can help to flush out toxins and excess fluids from the body. They also have anti-inflammatory properties, which can help to protect the kidneys from damage. Juniper berries can be consumed in the form of supplements, teas or can be used to flavor food.

Finally, ginger is another herb that is beneficial for kidney health. Ginger has anti-inflammatory properties and can help to reduce inflammation in the kidneys, which can help to protect them from damage. It can also help to lower blood pressure, which can help to prevent hypertension and kidney damage. Ginger can be consumed in the form of supplements, teas or can be used to flavor food.

In conclusion, there are several herbs that can be beneficial for kidney health. Dandelion, cranberry, cornsilk, parsley, juniper berries, and ginger are just a few of the many options available. However, it's important to note that while these herbs can be beneficial, they should not be used as a substitute for proper medical care and treatment. If you have kidney disease or are at risk of developing it, it's important to work with your healthcare provider to develop a treatment plan that is right for you. Additionally, it's important to note that some herbs may interact with certain medications or have potential side effects, so it's important to speak with your healthcare provider before starting any new herb or supplement regimen.

17

Supplements for Kidney Health

Supplements have become increasingly popular in recent years as a means of promoting overall health and wellness, and this includes the health of the kidneys. The kidneys are an essential part of the body's filtration system and are responsible for removing waste products and excess fluids from the blood. They also play a crucial role in regulating blood pressure, electrolyte balance, and the production of hormones that control red blood cell production and promote bone health. When it comes to kidney health, there are several supplements that have been found to be beneficial.

One of the most commonly used supplements for kidney health is omega-3 fatty acids. Omega-3 fatty acids are known for their anti-inflammatory properties, which can help to reduce inflammation in the kidneys. They can also help to lower blood pressure, which can help to prevent hypertension and kidney damage. Omega-3 fatty acids can be found in fish oil supplements, flaxseed oil, and other sources.

Another supplement that is commonly used for kidney health is magnesium. Magnesium is an essential mineral that is needed for proper kidney function. It helps to regulate blood pressure and electrolyte balance, which can help to prevent hypertension and kidney stones. Magnesium is also needed for proper bone health and can help to prevent osteoporosis, which is a common complication of kidney disease. Magnesium can be found in supplements, leafy greens and nuts.

Another supplement that is beneficial for kidney health is vitamin D. Vitamin D is essential for proper bone health and can help to prevent osteoporosis, which is a common complication of kidney disease. It also helps to regulate blood pressure and has anti-inflammatory properties, which can help to protect the kidneys from damage. Vitamin D can be found in supplements, fatty fish, egg yolks, and fortified foods.

Another supplement that is beneficial for kidney health is Vitamin C. Vitamin C is an antioxidant that can help to protect the kidneys from damage caused by free radicals. It also helps to strengthen the immune system, which can help to prevent infections that can damage the kidneys. Vitamin C can be found in supplements, citrus fruits and berries.

Another supplement that is beneficial for kidney health is N-Acetyl Cysteine (NAC). NAC is an antioxidant that can help to protect the kidneys from damage caused by free radicals. It also has anti-inflammatory properties and can help to reduce inflammation in the kidneys. NAC can be found in supplements.

Finally, another supplement that is beneficial for kidney health is alpha-lipoic acid (ALA). ALA is an antioxidant that can help to protect the kidneys from damage caused by free radicals. It also has anti-inflammatory properties and can help to reduce inflammation in the kidneys. ALA can be found in supplements, spinach, broccoli, and potatoes.

In conclusion, there are several supplements that can be beneficial for kidney health. Omega-3 fatty acids, magnesium, vitamin D, vitamin C, NAC and ALA are just a few of the many options available. However, it's important to note that while these supplements can be beneficial, they should not be used as a substitute for proper medical care and treatment. If you have kidney disease or are at risk of developing it, it's important to work with your healthcare provider to develop a treatment plan that is right for you. Additionally, it's important to speak with your healthcare provider before starting any new supplement regimen as some supplements may interact with certain medications or have potential side effects.

18

Stem Cell Therapy for Kidney Diseases

A Promising Approach for Targeting Damaged or Diseased Cells and Promoting Repair and Regeneration

Stem cell therapy is a promising approach for the treatment of kidney diseases. Stem cells are immature cells that have the ability to differentiate into various cell types, including those found in the kidney. They have the potential to repair or replace damaged or diseased tissue, making them a valuable tool for the treatment of kidney diseases.

One of the main advantages of stem cell therapy for kidney disease is its ability to target specific cells or areas of the kidney that are damaged or diseased. For example, stem cells can be used to replace lost or damaged renal epithelial cells, which are important for the proper function of the kidney. Additionally, stem cells can also be used to promote the repair and regeneration of damaged blood vessels in the kidney, which can help to improve blood flow and reduce inflammation.

Stem cell therapy has been shown to be effective in the treatment of various kidney diseases, including acute kidney injury, chronic kidney disease, and diabetic nephropathy. In animal models of acute kidney injury, stem cell therapy has been shown to reduce inflammation and promote the regeneration of damaged renal tissue. Similarly, in animal models of chronic kidney disease, stem cell therapy has been shown to improve kidney function and slow the progression of the disease. Additionally, in patients with diabetic nephropathy, stem cell therapy has been shown to improve kidney function and reduce the risk of developing end-stage renal disease.

There are several different types of stem cells that can be used for kidney disease treatment, including embryonic stem cells, induced pluripotent stem cells, and adult stem cells. Embryonic stem cells are derived from early-stage embryos and have the ability to differentiate into any cell type in the body. Induced pluripotent stem cells are adult cells that have been genetically reprogrammed to have the same properties as embryonic stem cells. Adult stem cells, on the other hand, are found in various tissues throughout the body and have the ability to differentiate into multiple cell types specific to the tissue they are found in.

The most commonly used stem cells for kidney disease treatment are mesenchymal stem cells (MSCs), which are adult stem cells found in bone marrow. MSCs have been shown to have anti-inflammatory and regenerative properties, making them well-suited for the treatment of kidney diseases. Additionally, MSCs can be easily harvested from the patient's own bone marrow, reducing the risk of rejection and making the treatment more accessible.

Another promising avenue of stem cell therapy is the use of stem cells to create organoids, which are three-dimensional structures that mimic the architecture and function of a specific organ. Organoids can be used to study the development and function of the kidney, and they have the potential to be used as a source of cells for transplantation.

However, while stem cell therapy holds great promise for the treatment of kidney diseases, more research is needed to fully understand the mechanisms by which stem cells promote the repair and regeneration of damaged kidney tissue. Additionally, the safety and efficacy of stem cell therapy for kidney diseases need to be further studied in larger, well-controlled clinical trials.

In conclusion, stem cell therapy is a promising approach for the treatment of kidney diseases. It has the potential to target specific cells or areas of the kidney that are damaged or diseased, and it has been shown to be effective in the treatment of various kidney diseases. However, more research is needed to fully understand the mechanisms by which stem cells promote the repair and regeneration of damaged kidney tissue and to ensure the safety and efficacy of stem cell therapy for kidney diseases in clinical trials.

19

Chapter 5

Managing and Reversing Chronic Kidney Disease

Preventing Kidney Disease Progression

Kidney disease, also known as renal disease, is a chronic condition that progressively damages the kidneys and impairs their ability to function properly. There are several lifestyle changes that can help prevent kidney disease progression and protect the kidneys from further damage.

One of the most important lifestyle changes that can help prevent kidney disease progression is maintaining a healthy weight. Being overweight or obese increases the risk of developing kidney disease and can also accelerate the progression of existing kidney disease. Losing weight through a combination of diet and exercise can help reduce the strain on the kidneys and lower the risk of kidney disease progression.

Another important lifestyle change that can help prevent kidney disease progression is controlling blood pressure. High blood pressure is a major risk factor for kidney disease and can damage the blood vessels in the kidneys, leading to a decline in kidney function. By controlling blood pressure through diet, exercise, and medication, individuals can help protect the kidneys from damage.

It is also important for people with kidney disease to limit their intake of protein. Too much protein can put extra stress on the kidneys, which can lead to kidney disease progression. It is best to consult a dietitian or a kidney specialist to determine the appropriate amount of protein intake.

Another key lifestyle change that can help prevent kidney disease progression is avoiding smoking and excessive alcohol consumption. Smoking damages the blood vessels and can lead to high blood pressure and other conditions that can harm the kidneys. Excessive alcohol consumption can also damage the kidneys, particularly over a long period of time.

Managing diabetes is also crucial in preventing kidney disease progression. Diabetes is one of the leading causes of kidney disease, and uncontrolled diabetes can lead to damage of the blood vessels in the kidneys, leading to kidney disease progression. By managing blood sugar levels through diet, exercise, and medication, individuals can help protect the kidneys from damage.

In addition to these lifestyle changes, it is also important for individuals with kidney disease to undergo regular check-ups and screenings to monitor their kidney function and detect any signs of progression. This can include blood tests, urine tests, and imaging studies. By detecting and addressing kidney disease progression early, individuals can take steps to slow or even reverse the progression of their condition.

In conclusion, kidney disease is a chronic condition that can lead to progressive damage to the kidneys, but there are several lifestyle changes that can help prevent kidney disease progression. These include maintaining a healthy weight, controlling blood pressure, limiting protein intake, avoiding smoking and excessive alcohol consumption, managing diabetes, and undergoing regular check-ups and screenings. By making these lifestyle changes and working closely with a healthcare provider, individuals can help protect their kidneys and preserve their kidney function for as long as possible.

20

Reversing Kidney Damage

A Multifaceted Approach

Reversing kidney damage, also known as renal failure, is a complex process that requires a multifaceted approach. The first step in reversing kidney damage is to identify and address the underlying cause of the damage. This may include managing and treating any underlying medical conditions, such as diabetes or hypertension, and making lifestyle changes, such as quitting smoking and reducing alcohol consumption.

Once the underlying cause of the kidney damage has been addressed, it is important to focus on maintaining and improving the function of the remaining healthy kidney tissue. This can be done through a combination of medication, lifestyle changes, and dietary modifications.

Medications that are commonly used to improve kidney function include ACE inhibitors, ARBs, and diuretics. These drugs help to lower blood pressure and protect the kidneys from further damage. Additionally, iron supplements and erythropoietin (a hormone that stimulates the production of red blood cells) may be prescribed to treat anemia, a common complication of kidney damage.

Lifestyle changes that can help to improve kidney function include maintaining a healthy weight, getting regular physical activity, and managing stress. A healthy diet that is low in sodium and high in fruits and vegetables is also important for maintaining kidney health.

Dietary modifications may include reducing protein and potassium intake. A dietitian can help to create a meal plan that is tailored to your individual needs. It is also important to stay hydrated by drinking plenty of water and limiting the intake of sugary drinks.

In some cases, kidney damage can be reversed through surgical procedures such as kidney transplant or dialysis. Kidney transplantation is the replacement of a damaged kidney with a healthy one from a donor. Dialysis is a procedure that uses a machine to filter waste and excess fluid from the blood.

It is important to understand that reversing kidney damage is a slow process and requires consistent effort and dedication. Regular monitoring and follow-up with a healthcare provider is necessary to track progress and make adjustments to treatment plans as needed.

In summary, reversing kidney damage requires identifying and addressing the underlying cause, maintaining and improving the function of remaining healthy kidney tissue through medication, lifestyle changes, and dietary modifications. In some cases, surgical procedures such as kidney transplant or dialysis may be necessary. Consistency and regular monitoring with a healthcare provider is crucial for success.

The steps for reversing kidney damage involve:

- Identifying the underlying cause: This includes identifying any underlying medical conditions, such as diabetes or hypertension, and addressing them through proper management and treatment.

• Making lifestyle changes: This includes quitting smoking, reducing alcohol consumption, maintaining a healthy weight, getting regular physical activity and managing stress.

• Medications: Medications such as ACE inhibitors, ARBs, and diuretics are commonly used to improve kidney function and protect the kidneys from further damage. Iron supplements and erythropoietin (a hormone that stimulates the production of red blood cells) may also be prescribed to treat anemia.

• Dietary modifications: A diet low in sodium and high in fruits and vegetables is important for maintaining kidney health. Reducing protein and potassium intake and staying hydrated by drinking plenty of water and limiting sugary drinks.

• Surgical procedures: In some cases, kidney damage can be reversed through surgical procedures such as kidney transplant or dialysis.

• Monitoring and follow-up: Regular monitoring and follow-up with a healthcare provider is necessary to track progress and make adjustments to treatment plans as needed.

It is important to note that reversing kidney damage is a slow process and requires consistent effort and dedication. It may take time to see significant changes, but with proper management and treatment, it is possible to slow down or even reverse the damage to the kidneys.

21

Improving Kidney Function: How to Protect and Support this Vital Organ

The kidneys are a vital organ in the human body, responsible for filtering waste and excess fluids from the blood. They also help regulate blood pressure, produce hormones, and maintain the balance of electrolytes in the body. When the kidneys are not functioning properly, it can lead to a variety of health issues, including kidney disease, hypertension, and anemia. However, there are several ways to improve kidney function and protect this important organ.

One of the most effective ways to improve kidney function is to maintain a healthy diet. A diet that is high in protein, fruits, and vegetables can help support kidney function, while a diet high in sodium, sugar, and processed foods can damage the kidneys over time. In particular, foods that are high in potassium can help to maintain healthy blood pressure and support kidney function. Additionally, maintaining a healthy weight and staying physically active can help to reduce the risk of developing kidney disease.

Another important step in improving kidney function is to control any underlying medical conditions that may be contributing to kidney damage.

For example, if you have diabetes or hypertension, it is important to work with your healthcare provider to manage your blood sugar and blood pressure levels. Additionally, if you have a family history of kidney disease, it is important to have regular kidney function tests to monitor your kidney health.

Medications can also play a role in improving kidney function. Some medications, such as diuretics, can help to reduce the amount of fluid in the body, which can help to protect the kidneys from damage. Additionally, some medications can help to reduce inflammation in the kidneys, which can also help to protect this important organ. However, it is important to work with your healthcare provider to determine which medications are appropriate for you and to monitor your kidney function regularly while taking them.

Another important step in improving kidney function is to limit your exposure to toxins and environmental pollutants. For example, exposure to heavy metals, pesticides, and other toxins can damage the kidneys over time. Additionally, smoking and drinking alcohol in excess can also harm the kidneys. By limiting your exposure to these toxins and making healthier lifestyle choices, you can help to protect your kidneys and improve their function.

Finally, it is important to be aware of the signs and symptoms of kidney disease, such as changes in urination, swelling, and fatigue. If you notice any changes in your kidney function, it is important to seek medical attention right away. Additionally, if you are at high risk for kidney disease, such as if you have diabetes or hypertension, it is important to have regular kidney function tests to monitor your kidney health.

In conclusion, there are several ways to improve kidney function and protect this important organ. By maintaining a healthy diet, controlling underlying medical conditions, taking appropriate medications, limiting exposure to toxins, and being aware of the signs and symptoms of kidney disease, you can help to improve your kidney function and protect your overall health. It is also recommended to seek medical help and advice if you have any concerns or symptoms related to your kidney.

22

Chapter 6

Coping with Chronic Kidney Disease

Chronic Kidney Disease (CKD) is a serious medical condition that not only affects the physical health of an individual but also has a significant emotional and psychological impact. Those living with CKD often experience a range of emotions such as anxiety, depression, and stress, which can make it difficult to manage the disease and maintain a good quality of life.

One of the most significant emotional impacts of CKD is anxiety. People living with CKD often have concerns about the progression of the disease, their ability to manage it, and the potential need for dialysis or transplant. Additionally, they may have fears about their ability to continue working or caring for their family, and the impact of the disease on their overall quality of life. This constant worrying can take a toll on an individual's mental well-being, making it harder to cope with the physical symptoms of the disease.

Depression is another common emotional response to CKD. People living with the disease may feel a sense of hopelessness and helplessness, which can lead to feelings of sadness, loss of interest in activities, and a lack of motivation. They may also experience feelings of guilt and shame, which can be exacerbated by the fact that many forms of CKD are caused by lifestyle choices such as smoking, drinking, and poor diet. Additionally, the physical symptoms of CKD such as fatigue and weakness can make it difficult for individuals to participate in activities they once enjoyed, further contributing to feelings of depression.

Stress is another psychological impact of CKD. The disease can be a constant source of stress, as individuals must manage symptoms such as fatigue, pain, and changes in their physical abilities. Additionally, they may experience stress related to the financial burden of the disease, as well as the physical and emotional toll of frequent doctor visits and treatments. Stress can also be caused by the fear of the unknown - not knowing what the future holds, and how the disease will progress.

CKD can also have a significant impact on an individual's relationships. The disease can cause physical limitations that make it difficult to participate in social activities and maintain relationships. Additionally, the emotional toll of the disease can make it difficult to maintain healthy relationships with family and friends. People living with CKD may feel isolated and alone, which can further contribute to feelings of depression and anxiety.

Moreover, the impact of CKD on one's body image and self-esteem can be devastating. People living with CKD may experience changes in their physical appearance due to weight loss, muscle wasting, and fluid accumulation. They may also feel self-conscious about changes in their skin color due to anemia, and about the smell of their breath due to uremia. This can lead to a negative body image and low self-esteem which can be detrimental to mental health and overall well-being.

In conclusion, CKD has a significant emotional and psychological impact on individuals living with the disease. Anxiety, depression, stress, relationship problems, and negative body image are common emotional responses to CKD. It is essential for healthcare providers to recognize and address the emotional and psychological needs of individuals living with CKD in addition to managing the physical symptoms of the disease. It is also important for family and friends of those living with CKD to be supportive and understanding of the emotional toll the disease can take. Mental health support and counseling can be beneficial for those struggling with the emotional and psychological aspects of CKD.

23

Navigating Chronic Kidney Disease

Support Groups and Resources Available to Improve Quality of Life

L iving with Chronic Kidney Disease (CKD) can be a challenging and isolating experience, but support groups and resources are available to help individuals manage their disease and improve their quality of life.

Support groups are one of the most effective resources for people living with CKD. These groups provide a safe and supportive environment where individuals can share their experiences, learn from others, and receive emotional support. They also provide an opportunity to connect with others who understand what they are going through, which can be especially beneficial for individuals who feel isolated or misunderstood by their friends and family. Support groups can be found in person, online or on the phone and can be specific to a certain stage of CKD or can be more general.

Another valuable resource for individuals living with CKD is education and information. Understanding the disease, its causes, and its progression is crucial for managing the disease and making informed decisions about treatment options. Many hospitals, clinics, and non-profit organizations offer education programs and informational materials for individuals living with CKD. Additionally, the National Kidney Foundation and the American Association of Kidney Patients are two national organizations that provide extensive information and resources for individuals living with CKD.

Nutrition and diet are important factors in managing CKD, and many resources are available to help individuals make healthy choices. Registered Dietitians (RD) or Certified Renal Dietitians (CRD) can provide personalized nutrition plans and guidance on how to manage dietary restrictions related to CKD. Additionally, many hospitals and clinics offer nutrition classes for individuals living with CKD.

Financial assistance is also an important resource for individuals living with CKD. The cost of healthcare and treatment can be overwhelming, and many organizations offer financial assistance and resources to help individuals manage the costs associated with CKD. The National Kidney Foundation, American Kidney Fund and the HealthWell Foundation are a few examples of organizations that provide financial assistance for individuals living with CKD.

Social workers, counselors, and psychologists can also provide support for individuals living with CKD. They can help individuals manage the emotional and psychological impact of the disease, and provide support and guidance for coping with the challenges of living with a chronic illness.

Lastly, Support from family and friends can be a significant resource for individuals living with CKD. They can provide emotional support, help with day-to-day tasks, and assist with transportation to medical appointments. They can also help educate themselves about the disease and ways to support their loved one.

In conclusion, there are a variety of support groups and resources available for individuals living with CKD. Support groups, education and information, nutrition and diet resources, financial assistance, mental health support, and support from family and friends can all play a vital role in helping individuals manage the disease and improve their quality of life. It is important for individuals living with CKD to seek out and utilize these resources as they work to manage their disease. It is also important for healthcare providers to inform and refer patients to these resources as appropriate.

24

Navigating Financial Assistance and Insurance Options for Managing Chronic Kidney Disease (CKD)

Chronic Kidney Disease (CKD) can be a financially and emotionally challenging condition to manage. The cost of treatment, medications, and doctor visits can add up quickly, making it difficult for some individuals to afford the care they need. Additionally, many individuals with CKD may be unable to work due to the severity of their condition, further exacerbating financial concerns. However, there are several insurance and financial assistance options available to help individuals with CKD manage the cost of their care.

One of the most important options for individuals with CKD is health insurance. Most individuals with CKD will require regular medical care and treatment, and having health insurance can help cover the cost of these expenses. Government-funded programs such as Medicaid and Medicare can provide coverage for individuals with CKD who meet certain income and eligibility requirements. Additionally, private health insurance plans may also offer coverage for individuals with CKD. However, it is important to carefully review the terms of the insurance plan, as some plans may not cover certain treatments or medications.

Another financial assistance option available to individuals with CKD is financial aid from non-profit organizations. Organizations such as the National Kidney Foundation, American Kidney Fund, and HealthWell Foundation provide financial assistance to individuals with CKD who are unable to afford the cost of their care. This assistance can be used to help pay for medical expenses, medications, and even travel costs associated with treatment.

Pharmaceutical assistance programs are also available to help individuals with CKD manage the cost of their medications. These programs are offered by pharmaceutical companies and can provide financial assistance or free medications to individuals who meet certain income and eligibility requirements. Additionally, some states have prescription drug assistance programs that provide financial assistance for individuals with CKD.

Additionally, patients with CKD who are unable to work may be eligible for disability benefits. Social Security Disability Insurance (SSDI) and Supplemental Security Income (SSI) are two government programs that provide financial assistance to individuals with a disability, including those with CKD.

Individuals with CKD may also be eligible for financial assistance through their state's Medicaid program. Medicaid is a joint federal and state program that provides health coverage to low-income individuals and families. Medicaid programs vary by state, but many states offer coverage for individuals with CKD who meet certain income and eligibility requirements.

Lastly, some employers offer long-term disability insurance to their employees, which can provide financial assistance to individuals with CKD who are unable to work. It is important to check if your employer offers this type of insurance and if you are eligible.

In conclusion, there are a variety of insurance and financial assistance options available to help individuals with CKD manage the cost of their care. Health insurance, non-profit organizations, pharmaceutical assistance programs, disability benefits, Medicaid, and long-term disability insurance are all options that can provide financial assistance to those in need. However, it is important to research and understand the different options available, as well as the specific requirements for each program. It is also crucial to work closely with your healthcare provider and financial advisor to ensure that you are getting the most appropriate and beneficial coverage for your specific needs.

25

Action Plan to Reverse and Manage Kidney Disease

1. Develop a Treatment Plan with Your Doctor: Create a detailed treatment plan with your doctor that outlines the best approach to managing your kidney disease. This should include diet and lifestyle changes, as well as medication or other treatments.

2. Follow Your Treatment Plan: Adhere to the treatment plan created with your doctor, including taking medications prescribed and making the necessary lifestyle and diet changes.

3. Get Regular Checkups: Make sure to get regular checkups with your doctor to monitor your kidney health and adjust your treatment plan as needed.

4. Exercise Regularly: Exercise regularly to promote healthy kidney function and reduce stress.

5. Eat a Healthy Diet: Follow a healthy diet that is low in salt and sugar and high in fiber and protein.

6. Reduce Stress: Make sure to take time to relax and reduce stress levels to help manage your kidney disease.

7. Educate Yourself: Learn as much as you can about kidney disease and how to manage it.

8. Seek Support: Join a support group or find a mentor to help you stay motivated and on track.

Conclusion

In conclusion, "The Kidney Disease Solution: A Comprehensive Guide to Managing and Reversing Chronic Kidney Disease" is a comprehensive and informative guide that provides a wealth of knowledge on the topic of chronic kidney disease. The book delves into the causes, symptoms, and progression of the disease, as well as the various treatment options and strategies available to manage and even reverse it.

The book presents a holistic approach that emphasizes the importance of a healthy diet and lifestyle, as well as the use of natural supplements, in managing and reversing kidney disease.

The book is a valuable resource for individuals with chronic kidney disease, those at risk of developing the condition, and their loved ones. It can help individuals take control of their health and improve their quality of life. Additionally, the book provides a clear and easy to understand language that makes it accessible to a wide range of readers. Overall, "The Kidney Disease Solution" is a must-read for anyone looking to better understand and manage this serious health condition.